Published By Adam Gilbin

@ Billy Tucker

Bulletproof Diet: A Recipe and Lifestyle Guide for
Lose Weight and Gain Maximum Energy the
Bulletproof Way

ISBN 978-1-990666-64-3

TABLE OF CONTENTS

Sweet Potato Smoothie

Ingredients:

- 1 1/2 cups coconut water

- 4 ice cubes

- 1 pinch cinnamon

- 1 large sweet potato, peeled and cubed

- 1 carrot, sliced

- 1/4 cup raw almonds

Directions:

1. Combine all the Ingredients: in a powerful blender or food processor.
2. Pulse for 1-2 minutes until smooth and well mixed.
3. Pour the smoothie in glasses and serve it right away.

Autumn Smoothie

Ingredients:

- 1 pinch cinnamon

- 1 pinch nutmeg

- 1 pinch ground star anise

- 1 sweet potato, peeled and cubed

- 1 cup butternut squash cubes

- 1/2 cup frozen cranberries

- 1 cup purified water

- 1 tablespoon MCT oil

- 1 cup coconut milk

Directions:

1. Mix all the Ingredients: in a blender or food processor and pulse until smooth and creamy.
2. Pour the drink in glasses and serve it as fresh as possible.

Bacon Maple Bulletproof Coffee

Ingredients:

- 2 tbsp sugar-free maple syrup

- Whipped cream for topping

- 1 bacon slice, cooked and crumbled

- 1 cup freshly brewed coffee

- 1 tbsp MCT oil

- 2 tbsp butter

- 1 tsp maple extract

- 1 tsp vanilla extract

Directions:

1. Add all the Ingredients: except the whipped cream and bacon to a blender, and process until smooth.

2. Pour the drink into a large glass, swirl some whipped cream on top and garnish with the bacon. Enjoy!

Mocha Bulletproof Coffee

Ingredients:

- 1 tsp unsweetened cocoa powder

- 2 tbsp swerve sugar

- 1 cup freshly brewed coffee

- 1 tbsp MCT oil

- 1 tbsp butter

Directions:

1. Blend all the Ingredients: until smooth and pour the drink into a glass.
2. Enjoy!

Winter Vegetable Salad

Ingredients:

- 4 tsp Bulletproof Brain Octane Oil

- 6 tsp Extra virgin olive oil

- 1 tsp Thyme, fresh

- 1 tsp Rosemary, fresh

- 1 tsp Oregano, fresh

- 1 pinch Sea salt (to taste)

- 1/2 small head Green cabbage (cored and cut lengthwise into 1-inch-thick slices)

- 2 tsp Apple cider vinegar

- 2 tbsp Almonds, raw (chopped)

- 2 thick slice Bacon (pastured)

- 227 gm Sweet potato (cut into 1-inch pieces)

- 227 gm Carrots (cut into 1-inch pieces)

- 227 gm Parsnip (cut into 1-inch pieces)

- 227 gm Winter squash (cut into 1-inch pieces)

- 227 gm Turnip (cut into 1-inch pieces)

Directions:

1. Preheat the oven to 320°F.
2. Line a baking sheet with parchment paper.
3. Arrange the bacon on the baking sheet and bake until just cooked through, but not browned, about 10 minutes.
4. Let cool and coarsely chop.
5. Reserve the pan and bacon fat and leave the oven on.
6. Add the vegetables to the bacon fat in the pan and toss with the Brain Octane oil, 4 teaspoons of the olive oil, the herbs, and salt to taste.

7. Bake until just beginning to soften, about 20 minutes.
8. Add the cabbage to the baking sheet, tossing to combine, and continue to bake, tossing once, until all vegetables are tender, about 30 minutes.
9. Drizzle the vegetables with the remaining 2 teaspoons olive oil and the vinegar and sprinkle with the bacon and almonds.
10. Serve warm or at room temperature.

Steamed Kale And Pineapple Smoothie

Ingredients:

- 1/2 avocado(s) Avocado

- 1 tsp Lime juice (fresh)

- 2 tbsp Whey protein powder, unflavoured

- 1 cup Kale (packed; centre stem removed; chopped)

- 1 cup diced Pineapple

Directions:

1. In a saucepan fitted with a steamer insert, bring a cup or so of water to a simmer.
2. Add the kale, cover, and steam until cooked, about 5 minutes.
3. Transfer the kale to a blender.

4. Measure out 1/4 cup of the steaming water and add to the blender along with the pineapple, avocado, and lime juice.
5. Blend until smooth and creamy.
6. Add more hot water if you want a thinner consistency.
7. For extra protein, add the protein powder and lightly blend until the protein is mixed in (optional).

Strawberry-Parsley Smoothie

Ingredients:

- 2 tablespoons avocado oil

- 1 tablespoon MTC oil

- 1 tablespoon vanilla upgraded protein

- ½ cup coconut milk

- 4 strawberries

- 1 bunch fresh parsley

Directions:

1. Place all Ingredients: in order into a food blender.
2. Blend until smooth and creamy.
3. Serve immediately.

Blackberry-Avocado Smoothie

Ingredients:

- 1 tablespoon coconut oil

- 1 tablespoon grass-fed ghee

- 10 ice cubes

- 1 cup blackberries

- ½ avocado, stoned, peeled

- 1 cup coconut milk

Directions:

1. Place Ingredients: in a food blender.
2. Process a few times or until smooth.
3. Serve immediately in a tall, chilled glass.

Salmon-Cuke Bites

Ingredients:

- Smoked salmon

- Cucumber, cut into ½ inch pieces

- Sea salt

Directions:

1. Cut the salmon into strips, and wrap each strip around a piece of cucumber (orzucchini or avocado).
2. Season with salt or salad dressing (as desired).

Shepherd's Pie

Ingredients:

- 1 c bone or veggie broth

- 2 heads cauliflower

- 1 c butter

- ½ lb. bacon, chopped

- 2 c shredded carrots

- 2 c diced celery

- 2 lbs. ground beef

Directions:

1. Cut and steam the cauliflower. Put it in a food processor or blender.

2. Add the butter and blend until nice and smooth. Set it aside.

3. Cook the bacon in a large fry pan, and then add the carrots and celery.

4. Continue cooking for about 5 minutes while you preheat the oven to 350 degrees F.

5. Add the ground beef to the fry pan along with a little salt and about half the broth.

6. Simmer and stir, adding more broth if it gets dry.

7. Cook until the broth has evaporated and the beef is cooked through.

8. Spread the beef mixture in the bottom of a large baking dish with high sides.

9. Spoon the cauliflower on top and smooth.

10. Bake uncovered for about 30 minutes until top starts to brown.

Bulletproof Smoothie

Ingredients:

- 1 tablesp of coconut oil, organic

- you can substitute coconut oil for the bulletproof branded oil

- 1 cup of organic coffee that has been brewed

- 1 tablesp of butter, use grass-fed only

- ½ of a cup of ice cubes

Directions:

1. Mix all of the Ingredients: together and make sure that the ice has been fully crushed.
2. There should be no large pieces of ice when you have finished mixing it up in the blender.
3. The ice should give it the appearance of a smoothie.

4. It will taste like a coffee smoothie and will give you the ice cold kick in the morning that you're looking for.

Vegetable Smoothie

Ingredients:

- 1 tablsp of peanut butter

- 1 tablesp of sugar free raspberry preserves

- 1 cup of ice cubes

- 1 cup of kale

- 1 tablesp of butter that is grass fed and organic

Directions:

1. Add all of the Ingredients: into your blender and mix up so that the ice is fully blended into the smoothie.
2. It will have a green tint to it but do not let that put you off.

3. It tastes exactly like a peanut butter and jelly without all of the guilt that comes with eating this often unhealthy snack.
4. You can substitute the raspberry preserves for a different fruit flavor.
5. You can also use any other super food vegetable that you want in the smoothie.

Coffee Smoothie

Ingredients:

- 1 tbsp. of coconut oil, organic can be used

- 1 tsp. of Stevia, or raw honey (Optional)

- 2 to 4 ice cubes

- 1 tsp. of organic gingerbread spice mix

- 1 tbsp. of grass-fed butter, or almond butter

Directions:

1. Combine the gingerbread spice mix with the Bulletproof Coffee grounds then brew the mixture.
2. Add the hot Bulletproof Coffee into a blender along with the remaining Ingredients:.
3. Use caution and blend the mixture until it is smooth.

Bulletproof Coffee Creamsicle Smoothie

Ingredients:

- 1 cup of ice, or less

- 2 ounces of organic orange juice, freshly squeezed

- 3 ounces of brewed Bulletproof Coffee, chilled

- 8 ounces of vanilla almond milk, or of choice

Directions:

1. Combine all of the listed Ingredients: into a blender and blend until the mixture is smooth.

Smoked Salmon And Eggs

Ingredients:

- ½ cup of salmon, smoked variety and wild caught variety

- 4 tablespoons of ghee, grass fed variety and fully melted

- 1 teaspoon of dill, fresh

- 4 eggs, pastured variety and poached

- Dash of salt, for taste

Directions:

1. First heat up your ghee in a large sized skillet placed over medium heat.
2. Once your ghee is fully melted add in your dill and cook for at least 30 seconds. Remove from heat.
3. Place your smoked salmon among two serving plates.

4. Top off with your poached eggs and cooked dill.

5. Season with a dash of salt and serve right away. Enjoy.

Delicious Hanger Steak With Herb Butter

Ingredients:

- 4 tablespoons of butter, unsalted variety and grass fed variety

- 1 tablespoon of chives, minced

- 2 tablespoons of oregano, fresh and roughly chopped

- 2 tablespoons of thyme, fresh and roughly chopped

- 2 tablespoons of rosemary, fresh and roughly chopped

- 1, ½ pound hanger steak

- 1 tablespoon of oil, mct variety

- 1 lemon, fresh, grated, zested and cut into halves

- Dash of sea salt, for taste

- 3 cups of spinach, fresh and roughly chopped

Directions:

1. Rub your steak with your MCT oil and set aside for later use.

2. Use a small sized bowl add in your fresh lemon zest, minced chives, fresh oregano, fresh thyme, fresh rosemary and dash of sea salt. Add in your fresh lemon juice and stir thoroughly to combine.

3. Next heat up a grill to medium or high heat. While your grill is heating up season your steak with your sea salt and place onto your grill. Red the heat to medium or low. Cook for the next 5 to 6 minutes on each side or until your steaks reach the desired doneness.

4. Remove your steak from your grill and allow to rest for the next 5 minutes.

5. Serve your steak topped with your spinach and freshly squeezed lemon over the meat. Enjoy while piping hot.

Bulletproof Chai Latte

Ingredients:

- ¼ tsp cinnamon powder

- ¼ tsp ginger powder

- 1 tsp sans sugar maple syrup

- 1 cup new emphatically prepared dark tea

- 1 tbsp MCT oil

- 1 tbsp unsalted butter

Directions:

1. Blend every one of the fixings in a blender until smooth and serv in a glass.

Herbal Bulletproof Coffee

Ingredients:

- 1 tsp MCT oil

- 1 tsp coconut oil

- 1 cup newly prepared natural coffee

- 1 tsp weighty cream

Directions:

1. Blend every one of the fixings in a blender and fill in a glass.

Basic Bulletproof Coffee

Ingredients:

- 3 tablespoons grass fed butter, unsalted

- 3 cups freshly brewed hot coffee

- 3 tablespoons Brain Octane or XCT oil

Directions:

1. Preheat the blender by pouring hot water into the blender. Discard the water.

2. Add all the Ingredients: into the blender and blend until a thick froth is formed on the top.

3. Pour into mugs and serve.

Flavored Bulletproof Coffee

Ingredients:

- Sweetener of your choice like, stevia, erythritol or hardwood xylitol

- 1 ½ teaspoons ground cinnamon / 1 ½ teaspoons vanilla / 3 teaspoons cocoa or 3 tablespoons dark chocolate

- 3 tablespoons Brain Octane or XCT oil or MCT coconut oil

- 3 tablespoons grass fed butter, unsalted

- 3 cups freshly brewed hot coffee

Directions:

1. Preheat the blender by pouring hot water into the blender. Discard the water.
2. Add all the Ingredients: into the blender and blend until a thick froth is formed on the top.

3. Pour into mugs and serve.

One-Pot Bulletproof Wonder

Ingredients:

- 3 cups water

- 3 tablespoons collagen

- ½ pound sweet potatoes, diced

- ½ pound carrots, sliced

- 1 zucchini, sliced

- 2 cups coconut milk, unsweetened

- 1 pound grass-fed beef chuck, diced

- Sea salt

- 3 tablespoons ghee, divided

- ½ inch ginger, sliced

- 1 tablespoon turmeric

- 1 tablespoon olive oil

Directions:

1. Apply salt directly to meat. On medium-high, heat 1-2 tablespoons of ghee in a large skillet.

2. As it bubbles, incorporate meat and cook in batches, allowing each side to brown slightly but not burn. (You do not have to thoroughly cook the meat in this stage - it will become cooked later.)

3. Add remaining ghee and ginger and stir for about 2 minutes.

4. Incorporate turmeric and stir for an additional minute.

5. Add water and collagen and let boil. Reduce heat to medium-low setting.

6. Cover and let simmer for 1 hour, stirring occasionally.

7. Incorporate vegetables and cook for an additional 15-25 minutes.

8. Incorporate coconut milk and olive oil before serving.

Bulletproof Fish Bake

Ingredients:

- ½ tablespoon ground turmeric

- ½ tablespoon oregano

- 1 tablespoon sea salt

- ½ pound wild-caught trout or tilapia

- 1/8 teaspoon vanilla powder

- 1/8 cup bulletproof-approved coffee beans, ground

- 1 ½ tablespoons hardwood xylitol

Directions:

1. Preheat your oven to 320° F.

2. Mix together first six Ingredients: and apply directly to the fish.

3. Bake until fish is thoroughly cooked.

Ground Beef Salad

Ingredients:

- 1/2 cup chopped red cabbage

- 2 cups spring greens

- 1 cucumber, sliced thinly

- 2 avocados, peeled and pitted ¼ cup apple cider vinegar

- ¼ cup freshly-squeezed lemon juice ¼ cup coconut oil, melted

- ½ cup cilantro, chopped

- 250 grams ground beef

- 1 tablespoon cayenne pepper

- 3 tablespoons fresh-squeezed lime water

- 2 tablespoons butter

- Pinch of salt

Directions:

1. Sauté the ground beef in a nonstick pan.

2. Cook beef for about 5 minutes or until cooked through.

3. Add the butter, cayenne pepper and lime juice to the beef.

4. Season the beef mixture with salt and then set aside.

5. Meanwhile, put the avocados, vinegar, lemon juice, cilantro and coconut oil in the blender; blend until the mixture is smooth and then set it aside.

6. Put all the vegetables and the beef in a large salad bowl.

7. Pour the avocado dressing over the salad and then toss to combine.

Easy Beef Casserole

Ingredients:

- 3 scallions, chopped

- 4 eggs, beaten

- Pinch of salt

- 250 grams ground pork

- 2 tablespoons coconut oil

- 2 large turnips

Directions:

1. Rinse turnips and pat dry. Peel them, grate them and then set aside.
2. Heat coconut oil in a pan and then cook meat until cooked through. Set aside to cool.
3. Add the scallions, turnips and eggs to the cooled meat.
4. Season with a pinch of salt and then mix well.

5. Transfer the mixture on a baking pan and bake at 400 °F for about 40 minutes.

6. Cover the baking pan with aluminum foil and bake for another 20 minutes.

7. Let the casserole cool before serving.

Delicious Paleo Donuts

Ingredients:

- ½ Teaspoon of vanilla extract

- 2 tablespoons of coconut oil

- 1 teaspoon of apple cider vinegar

- 2 eggs

- ¼ teaspoon of baking soda

- 3 tablespoons of pure maple syrup

- ¼ teaspoon of almond extract

- ¼ cup of unsweetened chocolate

- 2 tablespoons of coconut oil

Directions:

1. To begin with you will have to preheat the oven to 360 degrees Fahrenheit.

40

2. Grease your six mold donut pan with coconut oil.
3. After that, combine your dry Ingredients: into a medium bowl. In another bowl you should try to combine all the other Ingredients: and set up the egg whites.
4. It is now time to mix all the Ingredients: together and set them aside.
5. Beat the egg whites until they are nice and soft.
6. Gently fold the egg whites into the batter.
7. Equally distribute the batter between the six donut molds and smooth out the top of each donut.
8. You should bake the donuts between 12 and 15 minutes until they turn into a light golden color.
9. Allow the donuts to cool and remove them from the pan and let them chill in the refrigerator for about half an hour.

10. Place the glaze Ingredients: in a sauce pan and place the sauce pan into the skillet.

11. Gently mix the Ingredients: until they are fully melted.

12. Pour the melted chocolate into a bowl and gently dip each chilled donut into the chocolate.

Sweet Potato Bacon Cakes

Ingredients:

- 3 cups of flower

- ½ teaspoon of baking soda

- 2 cups of sugar

- 1 cup of butter

- 1 teaspoon of vanilla extract

- 1 teaspoon of cinnamon

- 2 teaspoons of baking powder

- 500 grams of sweet potato

- 2 eggs

Directions:

1. To begin with you will have to peel your sweet potatoes and then simply place them in a hot pan and cook them.

2. It is now time to use a bowl and add three cups of flour and two cups of baking powder.

3. You will also have to add one teaspoon of cinnamon and half a teaspoon of baking soda and ¼ teaspoon of salt.

4. It is now time to thoroughly mix all of the Ingredients:.

5. In another bowl you should add two cups of sugar and one cup of butter.

6. And mix them up. It is now time to add 1 teaspoon of vanilla extract and mix the Ingredients: really well.

7. After you mix all the Ingredients: you should add two eggs and continue to mix for a few minutes.

8. After you are done with mixing you can use another bowl to mash all of the potatoes.

9. You need to get them mashed really well and then add 2 cups of sweet potatoes to the mixture and mix it until it is nice and smooth.

10. Finally, you need to transfer the mix to your baking pan and bake at 350 degrees for 15 minutes.

11. In the end you should have your fast, delicious and easy to prepare sweet potato cake.

12. I really hope that you will enjoy this recipe as this is one of my all-time favorites.

Broccoli Pineapple Smoothie

Ingredients:

- 1 cup coconut water

- 1/2 cup coconut milk

- 1 pinch nutmeg

- 4 ice cubes

- 2 cups broccoli florets

- 2 slices fresh pineapple

- 1/4 cup cashew nuts, soaked overnight

Directions:

1. Mix all the Ingredients: in a blender, preferably a powerful one, and pulse until well mixed and smooth.

2. Pour the drink in glasses and serve it as fresh as possible.

Cucumber And Tangerine Smoothie

Ingredients:

- 1/2 teaspoon grated ginger

- 1 cup coconut water

- 1/4 cup almonds

- 1 tablespoon MCT oil

- 1 cucumber

- 1/2 cup fresh cilantro

- 2 tangerines, peeled

Directions:

1. Mix all the Ingredients: in a blender and pulse until smooth and creamy.

2. Pour the drink in glasses and serve it as fresh as possible.

Coconut Butter Bulletproof Coffee

Ingredients:

- 2 tbsp coconut butter

- 1 tbsp sugar-free maple syrup

- 1 cup freshly brewed coffee

Directions:

1. Blend all the Ingredients: until smooth and pour into a serving glass.
2. Enjoy!

Collagen Bulletproof Coffee

Ingredients:

- 2 tbsp collagen

- 2 tbsp butter

- 1 cup freshly brewed coffee

Directions:

1. Add all the Ingredients: to a blender and mix until smooth.
2. Enjoy in a glass.

Best Butter Beer

Ingredients:

- ½ of a teasp of butter rum extract

- 1 tablesp of your favorite grass fed butter

- 1 can of diet cream soda

Directions:

1. Melt your butter before you even begin because you are going to keep the cream soda cold the entire time (unless you like hot cream soda, then feel free to heat it up).

2. Mix the butter and the rum extract together to incorporate the flavor.

3. Slowly add the mixture to your cream soda and stir gently to avoid disturbing the soda and losing the carbonation.

4. You can also substitute this recipe for any soda, but it works best with diet cream soda, diet root beer, and diet birch beer.

Green Tea Smoothie

Ingredients:

- 1 tablesp of butter that is grass fed

- 1 teasp of vanilla extract

- 1 cup of ice cubes

- 1 cup of green tea, brewed to your preferences

- Juice from a single lemon

Directions:

1. Make sure that the tea has cooled off some and that it has steeped for your desired amount of time.
2. Do not heat your blender but add all of the Ingredients: that you have to the blender.

3. The ice should not be chunky and should be blended in with the rest of the Ingredients: so that it does not cause clumps.
4. Make sure that everything is blended the right way.

Nutritional Bulletproof Coffee Smoothie

Ingredients:

- 1 tablespoon of cocoa powder, unsweetened

- 1 sm. chopped organic banana, frozen

- 1 teaspoon of chia seeds

- 8 ounces raw organic milk

- 1 ounce of brewed Bulletproof Coffee, chilled

Directions:

1. Combine all of the Ingredients: into a blender and blend until the mixture is even and smooth.

Cold Brew Colada Bulletproof Coffee Smoothie

Ingredients:

- 2 ounces of regular water, or coconut

- 1 ½ teaspoon of hemp seeds

- 1 tablespoon of Stevia, or raw honey

- 1 cup of organic pineapple chunks

- 6 ounces of light coconut milk, or almond

- 2 ounces of brewed Bulletproof Coffee, chilled

Directions:

1. Combine all of the Ingredients: into a blender and blend until the mixture is smooth.

Hearty Asparagus Noodle Soup

Ingredients:

- 1 teaspoon of salt, for taste

- 1 teaspoon of black pepper, for taste

- 2 tablespoons of oil, coconut variety

- ½ teaspoons of rosemary, dried

- 1 lemon, fresh

- 1 pound of asparagus, fresh and trimmed

- 5 eggs, large in size

- 4 cups of beef stock, grass fed variety

- 2 cups of milk, coconut variety

Directions:

1. First slice your fresh and trimmed asparagus into small sized pieces.

2. Then heat up your coconut oil in a large sized soup pot placed over medium heat. Once your oil is hot enough add in your asparagus and cook for at least one minute.

3. Next add in your beef stock, coconut milk and dash of salt and pepper. Bring this mixture to a boil.

4. Once your mixture is boiling reduce the heat to low and cover. Allow to simmer for the next 20 minutes.

5. While your soup is simmering use a medium sized bowl and whisk your eggs until thoroughly beaten.

6. After 20 minutes uncover your soup and drizzle small amounts of your beaten egg into your broth. Allow to continue cooking for another 5 minutes or until your drizzled eggs are set.

7. Remove from heat and serve with a garnish of lemon.

Winter Style Vegetable Salad

Ingredients:

- 1 tablespoon of thyme, oregano and rosemary, fresh and roughly chopped

- Dash of sea salt, for taste

- ½ of a head of cabbage, small in size, cored and cut into thick slices

- 2 teaspoons of vinegar, apple cider variety

- 2 tablespoons of almonds, raw and finely chopped

- 2 slices of bacon, thick cut variety

- 2 ½ pounds of winter veggies like sweet potatoes, carrots and squash, cut into small pieces

- 4 teaspoons of oil, mct variety

- 6 teaspoons of olive oil, extra virgin variety

Directions:

1. The first thing that you will want to do is preheat your oven to 320 degrees.

2. While your oven is heating up line a large sized baking dish with some parchment paper.

3. Place your bacon on your baking sheet in a single layer and place into your oven to bake for the next 10 minutes or until thoroughly cooked through.

4. Remove and allow to cool completely before chopping coarsely.

5. Add in your vegetables with some bacon fat into a large sized baking dish.

6. Toss with your oil, olive oil, thyme, oregano and fresh rosemary and dash of salt for taste. Place back into your oven to bake for the next 20 minutes or until soft to the touch.

7. Add your cabbage to your baking sheet and toss again to coat in your bacon fat.

8. Place back into your oven to bake for the next 30 minutes or until all of your vegetables are tender to the touch.

9. Drizzle your cooked veggies with your remaining oil and vinegar.

10. Ass your bacon and almonds and toss to combine. Serve right away and enjoy.

Supercharged Coffee

Ingredients:

- 3 teaspoons MCT oil

- 3 tablespoons grass fed butter, unsalted

- 3 cups freshly brewed hot coffee

- 3 teaspoons red palm oil

- 3 teaspoons coconut oil

Directions:

1. Preheat the blender by pouring hot water into the blender. Discard the water.
2. Add all the Ingredients: into the blender and blend until a thick froth is formed on the top.
3. Alternately, add butter and oils into a bowl. Add coffee.
4. Steam for a while or place in a double boiler until it melts. Stir well.

5. Pour into mugs and serve.

Matcha Latte

Ingredients:

- ½ teaspoon chaga powder (optional)

- ½ teaspoon turmeric powder (optional)

- 2 tablespoons organic virgin olive oil

- 1 cup hot filtered water

- 1 cup coconut oil, cold or heated

- 1 – 2 teaspoons Matcha green tea powder

Directions:

1. Add all the powders to a small bowl.
2. Add a little hot water and stir into a smooth paste.
3. Add coconut oil and stir until it is well combined.

4. Transfer into a blender. Add coconut milk and blend until creamy.

Veggie Overload Side Dish

Ingredients:

- ½ tablespoon apple cider vinegar

- ½ teaspoon dill

- ½ teaspoon oregano

- ½ teaspoon sage

- ½ teaspoon thyme

- 1 cup asparagus, chopped

- 1 cup green beans, chopped

- 1 cup broccoli, chopped

- 3 tablespoons grass-fed butter, unsalted

- 2 tablespoons MCT oil

- Sea salt, to taste

Directions:

1. Combine vegetables and steam until they are tender but not mushy.
2. Blend together butter, oil, vinegar, herbs, and salt, and drizzle over vegetables.

Bulletproof Pesto

Ingredients:

- 3 garlic cloves, minced

- 2/3 cups high-quality olive oil

- 1/8 cup walnuts, finely crushed

- 1 cup basil, packed and chopped

- 1 cup spinach

- Sea salt, to taste

Directions:

1. Heat oil and garlic in a large skillet on medium.
2. Incorporate basil and spinach, and cook until vegetables have softened but are not soggy.
3. Serve with walnuts, and if desired, pair with cooked spaghetti squash.

Cauliflower Fried Rice

Ingredients:

- 80 Grams of onion

- 4 Tablespoons of water

- 200 Grams of frozen vegetables

- 50 Grams of bacon

- 200 Grams of cauliflower

- 30 Ml of liquid aminos

Directions:

1. This recipe is easy to customize and you can use any type of vegetable and any type of meat.
2. To begin with you will have to shred your cauliflower.

3. I would advise you to use a grader with fairly large holes as you need to make sure that the cauliflower is properly crumbled.

4. It is now time to heat the pan. After you heat the pan you might want to add in the chopped onion.

5. You will just want to saute it for a while. When your bacon is nice and crisp you know that it is time to add in the cauliflower.

6. Finally you should give a really good stir for about five minutes.

7. After you add the bacon you might want to add just a couple of tablespoons of water just so that the food is nice and steamy.

8. Let the cauliflower steam and add in any kind of vegetables that you may want.

9. It is now time to add the frozen vegetables.

10. I will add about half a bag of frozen vegetables and I will give it a good stir.

11. For the seasoning you can try to add fish sauce but my personal preference is liquid aminos.

12. I hope that you will give this recipe a try and I am sure that you will love this recipe!

Raw Vegan Ground Meat

Ingredients:

- 1 Clove of garlic

- ½ Cup of raw olives

- 4 Large button mushrooms

- ½ Teaspoon of cumin seed

- 2 Spoons of spice blend

- 2 Spoons of raw tomato ketchup

Directions:

1. To begin with you will have to make the raw tomato ketchup.

2. You may have to use a blender for this job but this is not mandatory.

3. After I finish with the tomato ketchup I am going to throw in my cumin seed and half of a tea spoon of garlic powder.

4. You can use any type of spice for this recipe, chili powder would also be great with this. I will also add in one clove of garlic.

5. After I finish adding all of the Ingredients: I am going to add three tablespoons of raw tomato ketchup.

6. You can use any type of blender that you want and the key is to blend it for at least 30 seconds.

7. You may not want to use it for more than 30 seconds because it will start to turn into a puree.

8. We will want this to be very grainy and meaty so we will just pulse it for a few times until everything gets blended together and forms a meaty texture.

9. If you want to give your meat a special taste you may want to add some nuts and seeds but these are only optional.

10. If you want your meat to have a stronger texture then you can mix the Ingredients: by hand.
11. This is the type of recipe that you can prepare early on in the morning.
12. It is really easy to prepare and the only downside of this recipe lies in the Ingredients: because you will have to take your time to select this wide range of Ingredients:.
13. Anyhow you can get this done in under 25 minutes and this is what I like the most about this recipe.

Mixed Berry Coconut Smoothie

Ingredients:

- 1/2 cup coconut water

- 1/4 cup coconut flakes

- 1 pinch cinnamon powder

- 1 cup blackberries

- 1/2 cup strawberries

- 1 cup coconut milk

Directions:

1. Mix all the Ingredients: in a blender and pulse until smooth.
2. Pour the drink in glasses and serve it as fresh as possible.

Fennel Carrot Smoothie

Ingredients:

- 2 pineapple slices

- 1 cup water

- 1 tablespoon lemon juice

- 1 small fennel bulb, sliced

- 2 carrots, sliced

Directions:

1. Mix all the Ingredients: in a powerful blender or food processor and pulse until smooth and creamy.

2. Pour the drink in glasses and serve it as fresh as possible.

Mushroom Powder Bulletproof Coffee

Ingredients:

- ¼ tsp cinnamon powder

- 2 tbsp butter

- 1 cup freshly brewed coffee

- 2 tsp mushroom powder

Directions:

1. Use a blender to mix all the Ingredients:.
2. Pour into a glass and enjoy!

Gingerbread Bulletproof Coffee

Ingredients:

- 1 tsp gingerbread spice

- 2 tbsp butter

- 1 cup freshly brewed coffee

Directions:

1. Add all the Ingredients: to a blender and mix until smooth.
2. Enjoy in a glass.

Bulletproof Cupcake

Ingredients:

- 1 pinch Himalayan sea salt

- 6 large egg Egg (pastured; room temperature; separated)

- 2 tsp Vanilla bean powder

- 1 tsp Cacao powder, raw

- 6 tbsp Erythritol

- 6 tbsp Xylitol

- 341 gm Dark chocolate chips (min. 85% cacao)

- 171 gm Butter, grass fed, unsalted (room temperature)

- 1 tbsp Sweet rice flour , Bob's Red Mill (see "Notes" below)

Directions:

1. Position racks in the upper and lower thirds of the oven and preheat to 350°F (180oC).

2. Line 20 cups of 2 muffin tins with paper liners.

3. Pulse the erythritol and xylitol in a blender until finely ground. Set aside.

4. In a small saucepan, bring about 2 cups of water to a simmer over medium-low heat.

5. Place the chocolate and butter in a large heatproof bowl that can sit on top of the saucepan but not directly touching the water.

6. Place the bowl on the pan and stir occasionally until the chocolate and butter are completely melted for about 10 minutes.

7. Remove from the heat and set aside to cool slightly.

8. In a stand mixer with the paddle attachment, beat together 6 tablespoons of the powdered erythritol/xylitol mixture, the salt, and egg

yolks on medium-high speed until the mixture is thick and pale, about 3 minutes.

9. Using a rubber spatula, gently fold the yolk mixture into the melted chocolate and stir in the vanilla powder, cocoa powder, and sweet rice flour.

10. In a separate bowl, with an electric mixer, beat the egg whites on medium speed until soft peaks form.

11. Slowly beat in the erythritol/xylitol, then increase the speed to medium-high and beat until medium peaks form. (Be cautious of erythritol's strongly cooling reaction with the proteins in the egg, which drops the temperature of the mixing bowl by about 20 degrees.)

12. Gently fold the egg white mixture into the chocolate mixture, one-third at a time, until combined.

13. Using a 1/4-cup ice cream scoop or cup
    measure, spoon the batter into the muffin
    cups.
14. Bake until a toothpick inserted in the center
    of a cupcake comes out with a few moist
    crumbs, about 25 minutes.
15. Let cool in the pan for about 5 minutes before
    transferring to a cooling rack to cool
    completely.

Avocado And Salmon "Not Sushi"

Ingredients:

- 114 gm Wild Atlantic salmon, smoked ("Sockeye")

- 1 pinch Sea salt, fine (to taste)

- 1 avocado(s) Avocado ("Hass")

Directions:

1. Cut avocado into 4 1⁄4-inch-thick slices; cut the salmon into four slices.
2. Wrap each piece of avocado in a salmon slice, and sprinkle with salt.

Celery-Lime Smoothie

Ingredients:

- ¼ cup fresh cilantro

- 1 apple, cored

- 1 tablespoon grass-fed ghee

- 1 tablespoon extra-virgin olive oil

- 1 cup filtered water

- 1 lime, peeled and seeded

- 3 celery stalks, chopped

- ¼ cup fresh parsley

Directions:

1. Place lime with celery, parsley and cilantro into a food processor.

2. Add remaining Ingredients: and process until smooth.

3. Serve immediately in a chilled glass.

Blackberry Cocoa Smoothie

Ingredients:

- 2 tablespoons cocoa powder

- 12 drops liquid stevia

- 2 tablespoons MTC oil

- 7 ice cubes

- 1 cup unsweetened coconut milk

- ¼ cup blackberries

Directions:

1. Place ice cubes in food blender.
2. Add remaining Ingredients: and blend it for 1-2 minutes or until everything is combined well.
3. Serve immediately.

Sweet Potato Ginger Brownies

Ingredients:

- 2 c cooked mashed sweet potato (purple ones if you can get them)

- 3 eggs

- ¼ c butter

- ¼ c raw honey

- 3 t coconut flour

- 3 t dark cocoa powder

- 2 tsp. Ground cinnamon

- ½ tsp. Ground ginger

- ¼ tsp. Vanilla powder

- ¼ tsp. Baking powder

- Pinch sea salt

- ½ c chopped lindt 90% dark chocolate bar

Directions:

1. Preheat oven to 350 degrees F.
2. Mix the mashed sweet potato with the eggs, butter, honey, and vanilla. Combine well.
3. Add in the coconut flour, cocoa powder, spices, baking powder, and salt.
4. Again mix well. Stir in the chocolate pieces.
5. Spread the batter in a buttered 8x8 pan. Bake 35-45 minutes until a toothpick comes out fairly clean. Cool before cutting.

'Whatever' Crock-Pot Dinner

Ingredients:

- 1 'green zone' meat

- 1-2 'green zone' vegetables, chopped

- spinach or kale

- your choice herbs/spices

Directions:

1. Put some coconut oil in a pan on medium heat.

2. Lightly brown the meat and then add the veggies and your leafy greens. Sprinkle in your spices and herbs.

3. Stir, cover, and cook on low for 6-8 hours.

Eggs Benedict

Ingredients:

- 1 small envelope of hollandaise sauce

- 1 tomato (optional)

- 2 eggs, poached

- 2 slices of lunch meat ham or Canadian bacon

Directions:

1. Poach your eggs or cook them anyway that you like.
2. You can also fry them in grass fed butter if you do not like your eggs to be runny at all.
3. Place the ham in a small pan with no butter to allow it to crisp for a few minutes.
4. Make your hollandaise sauce according to the Directions: .
5. Lay your pieces of ham on your plate.

6. Top with the tomato followed by eggs. Pour 1-2 tablespoons of your sauce over the top.

Cups Of Eggs

Ingredients:

- 1 bell pepper, cut similarly

- 1 onion, cut the same

- 2 eggs, mixed so they will scramble

- 1 slice of Canadian bacon or ham, chopped very small

Directions:

1. Heat your oven to 350 degrees.
2. Mix the onion, the pepper, the ham and the eggs together.
3. Grease a cupcake pan with organic cooking spray or use a silicone one to avoid doing that.
4. Pour the mixture into the cups.
5. One serving should take up about 4 of your muffin spots in the pan.

6. Cook for 15-20 minutes depending on how done you like your eggs.

Vanilla Bulletproof Coffee Smoothie

Ingredients:

- 1 teaspoon of raw organic milk

- ¼ cups of raw almonds

- 1 cup of ice, or less

- 1 cup of Bulletproof Coffee, chilled

- 5 organic dates, pitted

Directions:

1. Combine all of the Ingredients: into a blender and blend until the mixture is even and smooth.

Yummy Bulletproof Coffee Protein Smoothie

Ingredients:

- 1 tablespoon of raw honey

- 1 tablespoon of cocoa powder, unsweetened

- 1 scoop of chocolate protein powder, or of choice

- 1 cup of brewed Bulletproof Coffee, chilled

- 1 cup of ice

- 1 cup of almond milk, or of choice

- 1 chopped organic banana, frozen

Directions:

1. Gather all of the listed Ingredients:, add them into a blender and blend until the mixture is smooth.

Hearty Lamb Burger Salad

Ingredients:

- 1 red onion, thinly sliced

- ½ cup of tomatoes, cherry variety and cut into halves

- 1 cucumber, fresh and sliced thinly

- ½ cup of black olives, pitted and cut into halves

- 1 teaspoon of garlic, powdered variety

- 1 teaspoon of salt, for taste

- 1 cup of lamb, ground, lean and grass fed variety

- ¼ cup of oil, coconut variety

- 4 cups of salad greens, mixed

- 3 tablespoons of lemon juice, freshly squeezed

Directions:

1. First use a large sized bowl and add in your coconut oil, fresh lemon juice, half of your powdered garlic and half of your salt. Whisk thoroughly until smooth in consistency. Set aside for later use.

2. Use a separate bowl and add in your lamb, remaining salt and remaining powdered garlic. Stir to combine.

3. Form your lamb mixture into even sized patties. Place onto a preheated grill and grill for at least 8 minutes on each side or until completely cooked through.

4. Use a large sized salad bowl and add in your mixed salad greens, sliced onions, halved tomatoes, olives and sliced cucumbers. Toss to combine.

5. Pour your dressing over your salad and toss to combine.
6. Serve and top off with your grilled lamb burgers. Serve immediately and enjoy.

Delicious Steamed Pineapple And Kale Smoothie

Ingredients:

- ½ of an avocado, peeled and sliced thinly

- 1 teaspoon of lime juice, fresh

- 2 tablespoons of protein powder, optional

- 1 cup of kale leaves, fresh, packed and roughly chopped

- 1 cup of pineapple, finely chopped

Directions:

1. Use a medium sized saucepan with a steamer placed into it, add in a cup of water and bring to a simmer.
2. Once simmering add in your kale and cover. Steam for the next 5 minutes or until fully cooked through.
3. After this time transfer your kale to a blender.

4. Take at least ¼ cup of your steaming water and add it into your blender.
5. Add in your pineapple, fresh avocado and fresh lime juice.
6. Blend on the highest setting until smooth and creamy in consistency.
7. Pour into a large serving glass and enjoy immediately.

Vegan Bulletproof Coffee/Tea

Ingredients:

- 2 teaspoons to 4 tablespoons organic raw extra virgin coconut oil (depending on if you are new to this diet)

- Stevia to taste

- 1 teaspoon vanilla extract

- 2 cups freshly brewed organic coffee or chai or green tea

- 4 tablespoons coconut milk or almond milk

Directions:

1. Preheat the blender by pouring hot water into the blender. Discard the water.
2. Add all the Ingredients: into the blender and blend until a thick froth is formed on the top.
3. Pour into mugs and serve.

Vanilla Latte

Ingredients:

- 4 tablespoons grass fed butter, unsalted

- Stevia to taste

- 2-4 tablespoons coconut oil

- 4 cups hot water

- 2 teaspoons vanilla powder

Directions:

1. Preheat the blender by pouring hot water into the blender. Discard the water.
2. Add all the Ingredients: into the blender and blend until a thick froth is formed on the top.
3. Pour into mugs and serve.

Bulletproof Chocolate Ice Cream

Ingredients:

- 3 tablespoons grass-fed butter, unsalted

- 3 tablespoons coconut oil

- 2 tablespoons MCT oil

- ¼ cup chocolate powder

- 1 whole pastured egg

- 1 pastured egg yolk (used in addition with the aforementioned egg)

- 1 teaspoon vanilla powder

- 5 drops apple cider vinegar

- Ice

Directions:

1. In a blender or food processor, mix together all Ingredients:, with the exception of the water.
2. Keep blending until you have a creamy consistency.
3. Slowly add in a small amount of ice and continue to blend.
4. The texture should be smooth.
5. Then, pour the mixture directly into your ice cream maker to achieve ice cream consistency. Serve immediately.

Guilt-Free Cupcakes

Ingredients:

- Dash of sea salt

- 6 eggs, separated

- 2 teaspoons vanilla extract

- 1 teaspoon cocoa powder

- 12 ounces dark chocolate (must by 85% cocoa or darker), chopped

- ¾ cup grass-fed butter, unsalted

- 12 tablespoons hardwood xylitol

Directions:

1. Heat oven to 350° F. Prepare an 18 cupcake hole pan by lining holes with paper liners.

2. Use a blender to powder the xylitol (use the pulsing function for best results).

3. In a separate skillet, melt butter and chocolate on low, stirring constantly.
4. Remove from heat and stir frequently.
5. Mix half of the xylitol and egg yolks until you achieve a thick consistency.
6. Fold into chocolate and add vanilla and cocoa powder.
7. In a separate container, beat egg whites.
8. Use the "high" setting on your mixer and continue beating until soft peaks are able to be formed.
9. Incorporate them into the other mixture, folding in a small amount at a time.
10. Fill cupcake containers three-quarters of the way full and bake for 20-25 minutes.

Mashed Sweet Potato

Ingredients:

- 2 tablespoons sweetener

- Pinch of salt

- Pinch puff pepper

- 3 sweet potatoes

- ½ cup milk

- 3 tablespoons butter

Directions:

1. Rinse the sweet potatoes and then place them in a pot.
2. Cover them with water and then bring it to a boil.
3. Cook the sweet potatoes for about 10 to 15 minutes or until tender.

4. Remove the sweet potatoes from the pot and let them cool.

5. Peel the sweet potatoes and mash them using a fork. Set the mashed sweet potato aside.

6. In a saucepan, mix milk, sweetener and butter and then let it simmer for about 3 minutes.

7. Pour the mixture over the mashed sweet potatoes and mix well.

8. Season the mashed sweet potatoes with a pinch of salt and pepper.

Beef Steak Salad

Ingredients:

- 2 tablespoons freshly-squeezed lemon juice

- ½ cup cherry tomatoes, halved

- ¼ cup olives

- 1 clove garlic, minced

- 1 red onion, sliced thinly

- 4 cups romaine lettuce, torn into bite-size pieces

- 500 grams beef sirloin steak

- 3 tablespoons apple cider vinegar

- ½ cup coconut oil

- Pinch of salt

- Pinch of pepper

Directions:

1. Grill the steak for about 5 minutes per side and then set aside to cool.
2. When it is cool enough, cut it into thin slices. In a bowl, whisk coconut oil together with apple cider vinegar, garlic, lemon juice, pinch of salt and pepper.
3. In a large salad bowl, combine lettuce, onion, olives and cherry tomatoes.
4. Pour the dressing over the salad and toss to combine.
5. Top the salad with grilled steak slices and then serve immediately.

Very Berry Smoothie

Ingredients:

- 1/2 cup blackberries

- 1 cup coconut milk

- 1/2 cup strawberries

- 1/2 cup raspberries

Directions:

1. Combine all the Ingredients: in a blender or food processor and pulse until smooth.
2. Pour the drink in glasses and serve the smoothie as fresh as possible.

Pineapple Strawberry Smoothie

Ingredients:

- 1 cup coconut water

- 1 cup coconut milk

- 1/2 cup crushed ice

- 1 1/2 cups fresh strawberries

- 4 slices fresh pineapple

Directions:

1. Mix all the Ingredients: in a powerful blender or food processor and pulse until smooth and creamy.

2. Pour the smoothie in glasses and serve it as fresh as possible as it tends to lose nutrients in time.

Bulletproof Hot Cocoa

Ingredients:

- 2 tbsp unsweetened cocoa powder

- 2 tsp swerve sugar

- ¼ tsp cinnamon powder

- ½ tsp vanilla extract

- ½ cup coconut milk

- ½ cup filtered water

- 1 tbsp MCT oil

- 2 tbsp butter

Directions:

1. Boil the coconut milk in a pot over medium heat and pour into a blender.

2. Add the remaining Ingredients:, then blend
   until smooth and pour the mixture into a
   glass.
3. Enjoy!

Turbo Bulletproof Coffee Drops

Ingredients:

- ¼ tsp salt

- ½ tsp cinnamon powder

- 4 tbsp freshly brewed coffee

- 1 cup MCT oil

Directions:

1. Mix all the Ingredients: in a blender and pour the mixture into ice cube trays.
2. Freeze for at least 2 hours.
3. When ready to use, drop one or two pieces in hot coffee or water, stir and enjoy.

Bulletproof Coffee

Ingredients:

- 1 tbsp coconut oil (1 - 2 tbsp)

- 1 dash vanilla extract, pure ((optional))

- 1/2 tsp cinnamon ((optional))

- 2 cup brewed coffee (organic, fair trade)

- 1 tbsp butter, grass fed, unsalted (1 - 2 tbsp)

Directions:

1. Put all Ingredients: in a blender. Mix on high speed for 20 seconds until creamy and frothy.
2. Drink immediately while hot!

Raspberry Cabbage Smoothie

Ingredients:

- 1 tablespoon upgraded collagen

- 1 cup frozen raspberries

- 1 tablespoon lemon juice

- 1 cup shredded red cabbage

- 1 cup almond milk

- 1 tablespoon MTC oil

Directions:

1. Place all Ingredients: into a food blender.
2. Process until smooth and blended thoroughly.
3. Serve immediately.

Grapefruit Smoothie

Ingredients:

- 1 cup coconut milk, unsweetened

- 5 drops stevia

- 1 tablespoon upgraded XCT oil

- 10 ice cubes

- ½ cup pink grapefruit, sliced and chopped

- 3 celery stalks, chopped

- 1 tablespoon grass-fed butter

Directions:

1. Place ice cubes into a food processor.
2. Add remaining Ingredients: in order and process for 1-1 ½ minutes or until blended.
3. Serve immediately.

Bacon-Wrapped Cube Steak

Ingredients:

- 1 lb. Cube steak

- Sliced bacon

- Butter

Directions:

1. Fold the cube steak in half with a good-sized chunk of butter in the middle.
2. Wrap with bacon. Cook in a fry pan over medium heat until desired doneness, flipping from time to time.

Mean Green Bulletproof Coffee Smoothie

Ingredients:

- ½ cup of fresh spinach

- 1 cup of ice, or less

- 1 tablespoon of raw honey

- ½ tablespoon of coco powder, unsweetened

- 4 tablespoons of Bulletproof Coffee, chilled

- 1 cup of almond milk, or of choice

- 1 chopped organic banana, frozen

Directions:

1. Combine all of the listed Ingredients: into a blender and blend until the mixture is even and smooth.

Vanilla Brewed Bulletproof Coffee Smoothie

Ingredients:

- ½ cup of vanilla protein powder, or of choice

- ½ cup of raw organic heavy cream

- ¼ cup of raw organic yogurt, or of choice

- 2 cups of ice, or less

- 1 cup of brewed Bulletproof Coffee, chilled

Directions:

1. Combine all of the listed Ingredients: into a blender and blend the mixture until it is smooth.

Roasted Rack Of Lamb With Healthy Vegetables

Ingredients:

- 1 tablespoon of rosemary, fresh

- 1 tablespoon of turmeric, ground variety

- Dash of salt, for taste

- 2 cups of fennel, thinly sliced

- 2 cups of celery, fresh and thinly sliced

- 2 cups of cauliflower, fresh and thinly sliced

- 1 tablespoon of ghee

- 1 rack of lamb, fresh and grass fed variety

- 1 tablespoon of sage, fresh

- 1 tablespoon of thyme, fresh

Directions:

1. First preheat your oven to 350 degrees.

2. While your oven is heating up rub your ghee all over your rack of lamb.

3. Then season your lamb with your roughly chopped herbs and dash of salt.

4. Place your veggies into a large sized roasting pan. Place your lamb on top of your vegetables.

5. Place into your oven to bake for the next 45 minutes.

6. After this time turn your broiler to low and allow to broil for the next 5 to 10 minutes or until the skin is crispy.

7. Remove and serve whenever you are ready.

Lime Butter Smothered Rainbow Trout

Ingredients:

- ¼ cup of butter, grass fed variety

- ½ teaspoons of sea salt, for taste

- ½ teaspoons of black pepper, for taste

- 4 sprigs of rosemary, fresh

- 2 rainbow trout, wild caught variety, cleaned and with heads cut off

- ¼ cup of lime juice, freshly squeezed

- 1 lime, fresh and thinly sliced

Directions:

1. The first thing that you will want to do is preheat your oven to 320 degrees.

2. While your oven is heating up place your butter into a large sized cast iron skillet placed over medium heat.

3. Once your skillet is hot enough add in your fresh lime juice. Cook for at least one minute. Remove from heat.

4. Add your fish into your skillet and spoon your butter mixture straight into the trout bellies.

5. Add in your two sprigs of rosemary and season with a dash of salt and pepper.

6. Cover with some aluminum foil.

7. Place into your oven to bake for the next 30 to 35 minutes.

8. Remove from heat and serve with a few slices of lime. Enjoy.

Bulletproof Hot Cocoa

Ingredients:

- 4 tablespoons raw cacao powder or cocoa powder

- 4 tablespoons grass fed butter, unsalted

- ½ teaspoon ground cinnamon

- ½ teaspoon vanilla extract

- 1 cup full fat coconut milk

- 1 cup filtered water

- 2 tablespoons coconut oil or MCT oil

Directions:

1. Place a saucepan over medium heat.
2. Add water and coconut milk and bring to the boil.

3. Remove from heat and transfer into a blender.
4. Add rest of the Ingredients: and blend until smooth and frothy.
5. Pour into mugs and serve.

Bulletproof Chocolate Milk

Ingredients:

- 4 scoops vital proteins collagen peptides

- 2 teaspoons vanilla extract

- Stevia to taste

- Ice to serve (optional)

- 2 tablespoons ghee

- 3 tablespoon cocoa

- 2 cups coconut milk or almond milk

- 1/8 teaspoon salt

Directions:

1. Add all the Ingredients: to a blender and blend until smooth.

2. Pour into tall glasses and serve with ice if
    desired.

Best-Ever Guacamole

Ingredients:

- 4 ripened Hass avocados

- 1 tablespoon oregano

- 1 teaspoon freshly squeezed lime juice

- Handful fresh organic cilantro, chopped

- 2 tablespoons MCT oil

- Sea salt, to taste

Directions:

1. Hand-mix or blend Ingredients: until smooth.
    If desired, add a dash of vitamin C powder to
    prevent guacamole from turning brown.

Avocado Raspberry Smoothie

Ingredients:

- 1/2 teaspoon lime zest

- 1 cup coconut milk

- 1 tablespoon MCT oil

- 4 ice cubes

- 1 small avocado, peeled and pitted

- 1 cup fresh raspberries

- 1 teaspoon lime juice

Directions:

1. Mix all the Ingredients: in a blender and pulse until smooth.

2. Pour the smoothie in glasses and serve the drink as fresh as possible.

Chocolate Avocado Smoothie

Ingredients:

- 1 1/2 cups coconut milk

- 1 tablespoon erythritol

- 1 ripe avocado, peeled and pitted

- 2 tablespoons natural cocoa powder

Directions:

1. Mix all the Ingredients: in a blender and pulse until smooth and creamy.
2. Pour the drink in glasses and serve it as fresh as possible.

Bulletproof Gummies

Ingredients:

- 1 tbsp vanilla extract

- 5 tbsp gelatin

- 2 tbsp sugar-free maple syrup

- 1 cup freshly brewed coffee

- 1 tbsp MCT oil

- 1 tbsp butter

Directions:

1. Blend all the Ingredients: until smooth and pour into ice cube moulds
2. Chill in the fridge until firm and enjoy as a snack.

Bulletproof Green Tea

Ingredients:

- 1 tbsp heavy cream

- ½ cup ice cubes

- 1 cup freshly brewed green tea

- 2 tbsp MCT oil

- 2 tbsp butter

Directions:

1. Blend all the Ingredients: until smooth and fill into a glass.
2. Enjoy!

Bulletproof Elixir

Ingredients:

- 1 heaped tablespoon chia seeds

- ½ tablespoon cacao powder

- ½ teaspoon vanilla powder

- 10 stevia drops

- 2 tablespoons upgraded vanilla protein powder

- 1 cup warm green tea

- 1 tablespoon coconut oil

- 1 tablespoon grass-fed butter or ghee

Directions:
1. Place all Ingredients: into a food blender.
2. Process until smooth and creamy.

3.   Serve immediately in a chilled glass.

Banana Radish Smoothie

Ingredients:

- 2 radishes, washed, sliced

- 2 tablespoons grass-fed ghee

- 1 tablespoon upgraded collagen

- ½ cup unsweetened coconut milk

- 1 medium banana

- ¼ cup ice

Directions:

1.   Place ice cubes into a food blender.
2.   Add banana and radishes.
3.   Process until smooth; add remaining
     Ingredients: and process until frothy and
     blended well.

4. Serve immediately.

Pancakes

Ingredients:

- 1 teasp of cinnamon

- 1 teasp of vanilla

- 2 eggs

- 1 banana

Directions:

1. Blend your eggs, the banana, and your flavors together into a blender.
2. Do not heat the blender before you make the mixture.
3. Heat a medium sized pan until droplets of water dance on it when they are put in the pan. Pour your mixture in and cook.
4. Flip only when there are bubbles on top of the mixture to avoid undercooking the pancakes

and to make sure that you are able to truly flip them.

5. Make smaller pancake medallions to make it easier for you to flip them.

Bread For Butter

Ingredients:

- ½ of a block of cream cheese

- A small pinch of salt

- 3 large eggs that have been separated

Directions:

1. Heat your oven until it is 350 degrees.

2. Make sure that there are no yolks in with your egg whites and whip the egg whites until they form peaks, like if you were making a meringue.

3. Mix the cream cheese once it is soft with the yolks of the eggs.

4. Mix it up only until it is blended and not any more than that because it may not be as good.

5. Gently combine the two bowls to make the batter.
6. Spoon the batter onto a greased baking sheet.
7. Bake for around 10 minutes depending on the type of sheet you have and the oven that you have.
8. Spread with grass fed butter or sugar free preserves.